The Lice Program
(*Be free of head lice in 21 days*)

by

Mol Smith

ONVIEW BOOKS
The Lice Program
(*Be free of head lice in 21 days*)
by
Mol Smith

Published by Onview.net Ltd
In association with www.createspace.com
2015

Onview.net Ltd. Registered Office:
Frilford Mead, Kingston Road, Frilford. Abingdon.
Oxfordshire. OX13 5NX England

www.onview.net

First Published 2015 by (Onview Books) Onview.net Ltd.
In association with www.createspace.com

A CIP catalogue record for this book is available.

ISBN-13: 978-1508849353
ISBN-10: 1508849358

The Lice Program
(*Be free of head lice in 21 days*)

by

Mol Smith

"Know your enemy!"

CONTENTS

Chapter 1: Introduction

I know you will probably want to get started right away to get rid of those pesky head lice (also called hair lice), but it's worth just getting acquainted with me, the author, and why this book, and this program is finally going to work. Probably everything else you tried failed already, and now you are falling into thinking nothing is ever going to get rid of the lice.

Wrong.

I will. I need a little help from you though. So, let's say—*we* will!

I think it's important you have faith in me. I am not one of those annoying sales persons, or someone behind a web site (you know the type—all cleverly done to make you buy this thing or that thing). You can google me: 'mol smith'. I run a microscopy site. I write books. I make films. I put the Lice Program, free for all, on www.microscopy-uk.org.uk. Check me out. I'm a good guy. I help others, I spread good information. I'm not rich, but I love life, so I don't need to be. I could be, but I love other aims more than focusing on money. We'd all like more, I'm sure, but I have enough for my needs and it's probably a lot more than most folk have so why should I want more?

My reason for producing this book is simple. I know how to do it. So, why not? You have paid a small amount for this book, and sure, I get some of that. It'll probably be spent on doing more to advise or help others. And I know it is cheaper and more effective than anything else you will have tried.

What has happened to you, or your children, or loved one happened to me. So I know how you feel. The one big difference is those ugly blood-sucking parasites happened to infect the family home of a guy in London, England, who was also interested in science and owned a microscope. More, that guy (yup... me) also hosted a very successful internet web site aimed at supporting people interested in studying tiny organisms with a microscope.

My wife and my young daughter both became infested with head lice, and just like you, we did it all: the lotions and potions, the combing, hair-washing, bed sheet washing etc. etc. None of it worked!

I don't like to be beaten by anything. And I certainly didn't like my pretty young daughter being bothered by having minute parasites crawling over her head, sucking her blood whenever they wanted to. What did I do? I researched and studied them properly. I looked at books from the past by people who lived in Victorian London and studied these things like no one else ever has before.

I set up a small glass tank, put hair in it, caught some lice and put them in. I fed them daily with my blood so I could keep them alive and learn their life cycles and breeding habits. I tried to kill them directly using lotions purchased from the drug store designed to do just that—eradicate them. I poured the stuff on them. They 'laughed ' at it. None of the lotions worked. I contacted the people (the company) who made the stuff) and sent them videos I had made of pouring their useless product over the lice and showing they carried on living.

And then I sat down and worked out exactly what was going on and why we all end up running around infested when our kids are young and at school, and why we stay infested despite shelling out hard earned money on products that do not do what they say on the bottle.

What we are going to use to kill them is the one thing humans have above all other creatures: our intelligence. I'm going to arm you with the insight I have and knowledge from the study I have done, and I'm going to do that so it's easy to understand. Once you know it, I'm going to let you loose for 3 weeks on your own to wreak havoc on the lice enemy and wipe them out of your life, and then you will love me forever because those darn mini-monsters are gone.

I think if I were to give you a gun and expect you to go and kill a load of monster blood sucking beasts, I would not have done my job until I had also taught you how to aim and shoot, when to duck, and how to win your war. It's the same here with guiding you through your war and winning it over the head lice. It won't take long, but an informed you is better than an un-informed you, if you are resolved to get rid of the lice. So, let's get going...

Know Your Enemy

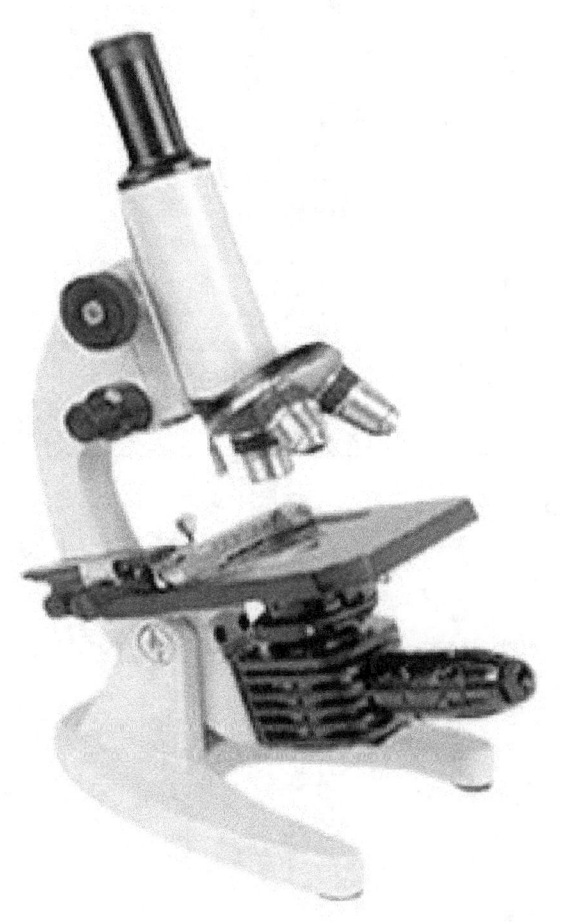

Chapter 2: Know Your Enemy

There are three types of lice which infest humans. The most widespread and commonest type is the one we commonly call the **head louse**.

YES!

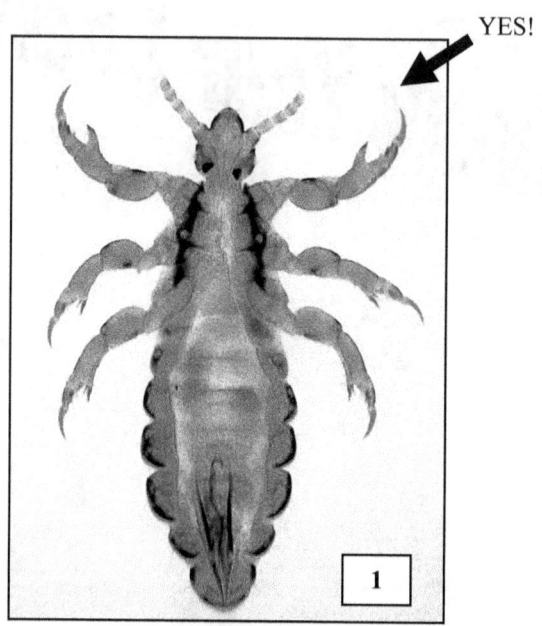

1. HEAD LOUSE

NO!

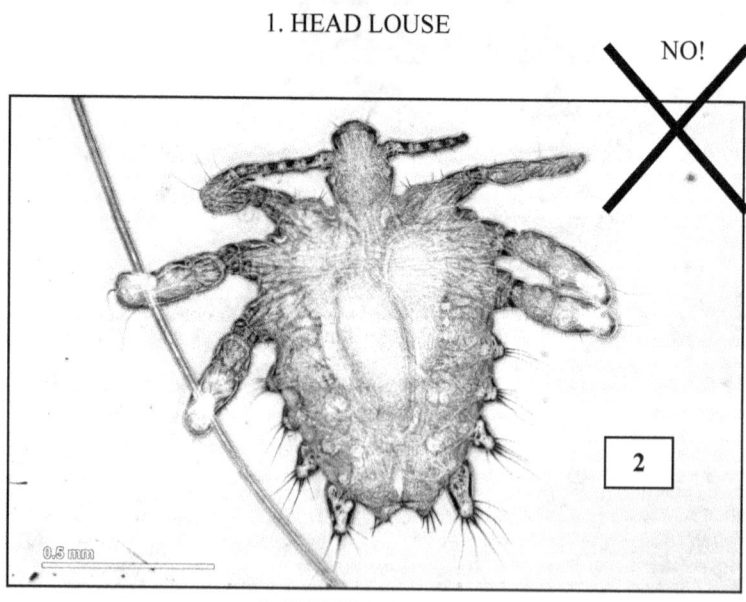

2. PUBIC LOUSE

You are only concerned with this one. The other two types [2] the pubic louse and [3] the body louse can not live on a human head, nor in human head hair. The pubic louse lives in the pubic area of the body in infested people. It is normally transmitted from one person to another via sexual activity, and close body parts.

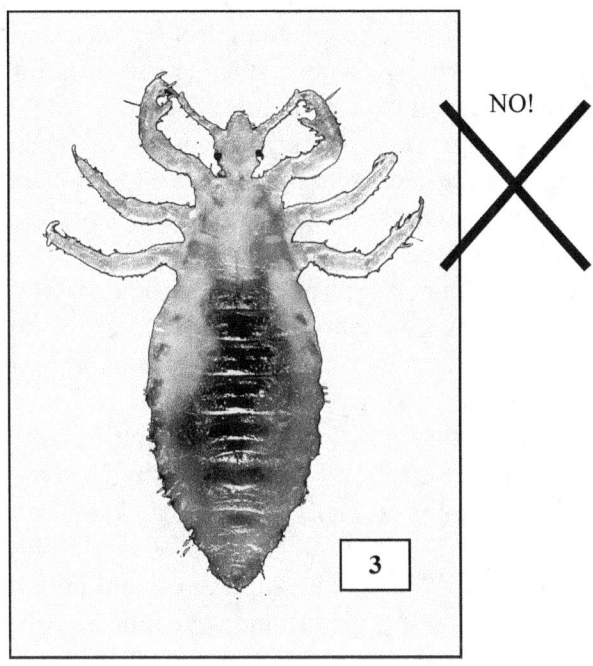

3. BODY LOUSE

It is commonly the thing people speak of when (if) they confess they have 'crabs'. No matter what you or anyone else might say—these cannot live on your head (no matter what kind of sexual activity an adult might get up to). Their body structure and design is completely dedicated to activities it carries out in the pubic area.

The third type of louse, less common today in the western world is the body louse [3]. In truth, these live in clothes and pop onto the human only for a feed. They are designed to travel around the fibres of articles of clothing we wear close to our skin. Once again, these body lice cannot live on a human head, even if you stuck your head into an infested item of clothes. Sure, they might climb onto your head, but they cannot survive long there and will just die.

Now, I could give you the Latin names for these three lice, but unless you are studying to be a medic, doctor, or something like that, you don't need to know. You just need to understand a bit about one of them—the HEAD Louse. These critters have been with us for a very long time, probably back to the beginning of our time on earth. No wonder they are so difficult to get rid of, eh? The main reason we find them difficult to kill is because they evolve and adapt very quickly. A drugs company brings out something designed to kill them, and indeed it works... for a while. But what happens is in many thousands of lice, there will always be one less affected by whatever new poison comes along. It might live longer before being killed or not die at all. Ultimately, a new generation of drug resistant head lice emerge into our lives, and we go on buying the same old poisons from the drug store but they no longer work!

Over our human lives, it seems infestations come in waves, reaching a peak, subsiding, and then rising again—a few years later. This is due to the evolving louse and the 'catching up' by drug companies. And all of this is a big problem for drug companies. To kill the things walking around on your head, they have to invent a new poison, and that poison will be absorbed through your scalp and pass into you too. They have to make sure the poison, in the small doses absorbed by you, are not going to harm you. The process takes many years.

The result of this time lag ends up with the fact there is always a period when a new evolved head louse is around (a SUPER LOUSE) and there is nothing out there available to kill it. And it doesn't matter how clean you keep yourself or your child. Lice love 'clean'. They love the natural oils of your hair and scalp. It nurtures them. Without the oils your body creates and pushes up through your scalp, they dry out and die! It is not just your blood they need. They need your warmth, the oils you produce, and the hair on your head to travel easily around on.

They move rapidly and switch from hair to hair with the ease of a trapeze artist. But if they are not in your hair, they can hardly move at all. It's like one of us walking around on our elbows and knees—instead of on our feet. They need those claws in your hair. So, if they fall off and get on the floor or onto towels with thicker fibres than your hair... or they fall onto the sheets or pillow or duvets, or the floor... they have had it!

So, there is little point washing bed linen, or clothes, thinking it will help you get rid of them. You'll be wasting your time because all that is unnecessary. We don't need to waste time and energy doing that one.

They can survive under water too. You can stick your head under the water as long as you like, they'll still be there when you pull it out again. And they'll still be alive. Formidable foes indeed! But they are not bright like us. Washing your hair or your children's hair over and over again is not going to achieve anything. It is just more wasted effort. Our lives, especially when we have a family, kids, and jobs to do is more than enough to cope with. We are not super-human.

The first thing to do is save time and focus it where it is most effective. The second thing to do is to understand that although hair lice are a nuisance (and not nice), they do not spread any infection, disease, and will not harm you or your child in any way. We don't have to panic. We can be focused. We can outwit them.

We don't want to waste money on this chemical or that remedy, or anything which is sold to fix the issue, because some of that works sometimes, and other times it doesn't. Remember, the people making the remedies cannot keep up with the rate of evolution and how rapidly new chemical-resistant species of hair lice appear.

We are going to apply real focus over the minimum amount of time and with no wasted effort or disruption to our family lives. We are going to understand how one pair of lice start up, keep going, grow to maturity and lay eggs. We can't get rid of eggs. The lice stick them to hair shafts with a glue better than super-glue. We don't need to remove the eggs. We want them to hatch. Then we can remove the hatchlings, the new generation of lice, before they become mature enough to have sex with each other and lay new eggs. We don't have to kill anything. We don't need chemicals on heads, our kids heads, killing with poison. We are smart. Chemicals do not always work. 'Smart' always works if we are smart enough.

Lice have a fantastic and almost fool-proof way of reproducing and laying new eggs. It is (if you wish) the reason for their success. But, once you know this, it is also their weakness. It is far easier for them to adapt and evolve to resist our various chemical weapons against them than it is for them to alter their time-tested and proven reproduction methods.

And that is where we come in. We are going to remove all the egg laying mature females. We are going to remove all the seeding mature males. And then we are going to sit back and wait for the eggs to hatch. When they do, we are going to remove all the new baby lice There will be nothing left to breed or lay eggs. They are all gone!

This will take 21 days.

I wish it was 3 days, but it isn't. It has to be 21 days because that is the time for the cycle of events taking place in their lives—the lice. And we are going to eradicate them by disrupting them at their weakest point. It is actually their strongest attribute but not now we know of it.

It is not something you will be doing for very long. Maybe an hour a day. I call it the Lice Program. You have to do it just the way it is designed. If you miss one small point, it may work and maybe it won't. But if you miss nothing, it will.

This is what a program is. A set of rules and actions to be performed precisely no matter what else we have to do to keep our lives and our show on the road. It doesn't hurt. It brings the family together for an hour or so most days. It takes 3 weeks. And the outcome is 100% certain.

Once you are free of head/hair lice, you need to stay free, but we can talk about that later.

Let's get started on the program...

Chapter 3: Destroying Success

How do you destroy the success of something which has been going on for thousands of years? You find out why the success is happening. You look at the stages of each step which leads to success. You look for the one tiny thing you can do to interrupt that step, and then you interrupt it.

Lice succeed because of a pattern of time. We do also. We get up at the same time to go to work. We feed our kids in a routine pattern of time, or catch a bus, train, or drive to work. We do it over and over again. But when something goes wrong... a flat tyre one morning, a late bus. What happens? Trouble! And if it keeps happening, if the bus keeps coming late, or every morning the tyre is flat.. bigger trouble. Goodbye job!

Lice are no different. They take time to grow. Time to mate. Time to hatch. Time to die. The secret of their success comes down to 21 days.

To get rid of lice, you need to remove all lice in your hair from all hatched eggs and have no eggs left in your hair waiting to hatch.

The complete life cycle of the head louse is:-
Egg stage: 7 days (it can vary 5 - 10 days)
Larva: 4 days
1st Nymph: 3 days
2nd Nymph: 2 days
Pre-egg-laying adult stage: 1 day
Egg Laying adult: 30 days (Life span).

The important fact is there are 17 days in the egg-laying cycle. This means from the first egg being laid to the next generation egg being laid is approx. 17 days. It can be as short as 15 days and as long as 20 days. So... 21 days to be 100% certain!

Now the important bit is this: not all eggs get laid at the same time, and they do not hatch at the same time. There are spans of days over which each incident happens. So, imagine you have a 100 fertilised chicken eggs sitting out there in your garden, or a spare room. Let's say you can't damage the eggs. They are made of steel. Let's also say you can't move them either: someone glued them there with a glue which is super-super glue. You don't want chickens. What you have to do is get out there and as they hatch, take them, the new chickens—and chuck them away somewhere else. But you don't have time to go where the eggs are every day. And if you can't get there in a regular kind of way, you know some of the eggs will hatch, and before you get there to remove the little ones, they've grow up enough to mate with each others and lay new steel, glued down eggs. It's a nightmare! Before long, you will be grabbing hold of chickens and chucking them out and each time you go back... more flipping chickens! Maybe you can get something to destroy the eggs? You can't. Whatever was made to do that, doesn't work on these eggs.

This is what you have been doing. And this is why the lice problem drives everyone mad!

But supposing there was a moment or maybe two moments when all the eggs have hatched and all the chickens are out of the shells running around, but so far none of them can mate. If you got to them then and chucked them out... no more chickens! But you never know which day that is because it varies. But then someone tells you the days when it varies. So you just have to get there those few days and whip out all the chickens.

This is what we are going to do with the lice. Exactly that. Ready? We need to prepare. We need to get our timing right. We need to agree a day with all the family so we are all synchronised and committed. One moment missed, and we've blown it.

So, get a calendar, talk to the others, mark a day in the calendar, and make sure everyone in the house knows that day. No excuses then about anyone not being available in the 3 weeks which follow it. This might seem a bit excessive! But how long do you want to be going on thinking you got rid of something and then, as if by magic, a few weeks later (sometimes a month or more)... the lice are back. I know. I did all that too! The thing is you never got rid of them in the first place. You think you did. But you didn't. You just reduced the numbers so it took a while before they mated and grew their number to such an extent that you noticed them again. This is not going to happen this time. *Set a date in the calendar.*

You need a weapon too. You need it ready for the day. It doesn't cost much, but you are going to have to buy it. You don't want a cheap, doesn't work kind of one. You want a well made one which has been designed and made properly. It's not so much a weapon. It's more like a great shovel. It's called a lice comb! You are going to use it to scoop out the lice and throw them away. This is going to be your only tool. It is the thing you will come to rely on. Cheap is plastic. Cheap is something called a lice comb, looks like a lice comb, but isn't a lice comb. It is a pile of rubbish. A good lice comb is like a pencil you write with that doesn't break it's lead... or a pencil that when you sharpen it, the lead doesn't fall out. It is a simple thing but so simple, everyone thinks they can make one and sell it to you, and you won't sue them when it doesn't work.

Most pencils don't work like you expect them to work anymore. So it is with lice combs. Good ones cost a few cents or pennies more than a bad one. Everyone sells the bad ones because the profit-mark-up is good. But you are going to commit 3 weeks to get rid of lice. And you don't really want to spend that kind of commitment and waste it on relying on a cheaply-made looks-like-a-lice-comb pile of sh..i... (er)...   rubbish! You need something which will not cost much, but actually works. I don't sell lice combs. And you live in a different place to me. So I am going to tell you the lice comb you need to buy and you can seek it out. I am not connected with this kind of lice-comb selling company or that one. I have bought several over the years and looked at how they are made. You are free to pick you own from an internet-buy or at a local store. But this is what you need...

The Lice Comb
A lice comb is a fine toothed comb with very tiny gaps between long teeth. Several different types exist, from fancy to simple. Some are plastic and some are metal. We only want a plain, simple, metal lice comb. Plastic ones are no good. The teeth tend too bend at the tip or separate allowing the louse to escape. We don't want a cheap metal one either. The teeth have to be strong to prevent them being pushed away from each other and creating wide gaps for the lice to escape being combed out. A typical good, metal, lice comb will cost about £6.00 ($9.50) on line. Don't buy anything else. You don't need it.

Here are two types of metal combs. You need to buy one of these.

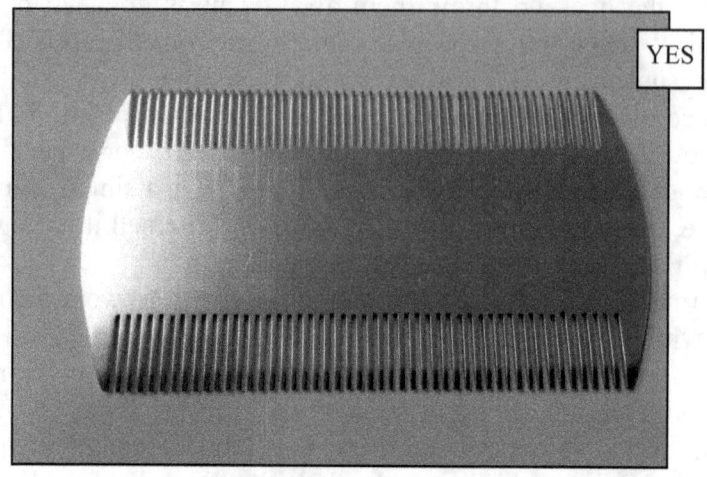

YES

YES. METAL COMB. WE WANT THIS ONE!

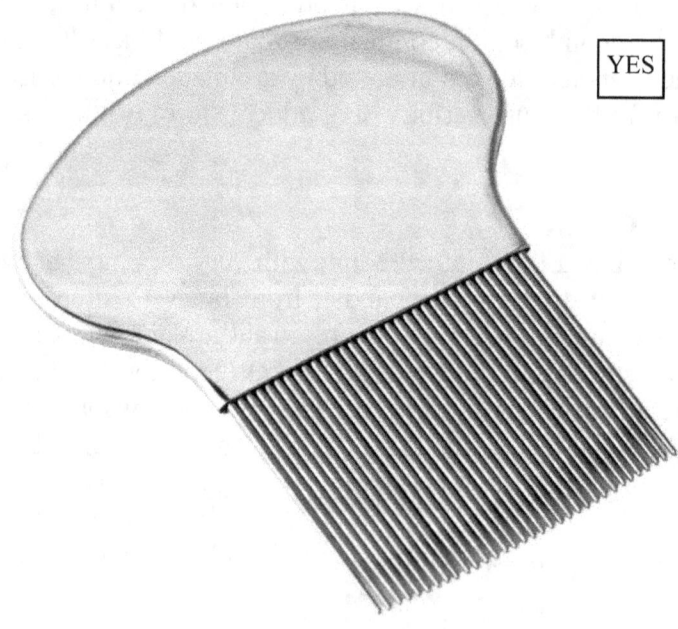

YES

YES. METAL COMB. WE WANT THIS ONE!

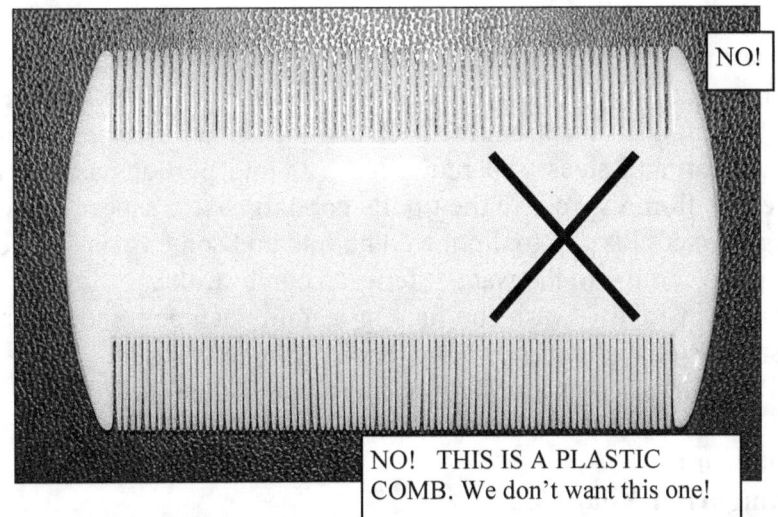

NO!

NO! THIS IS A PLASTIC COMB. We don't want this one!

Using The Comb Properly

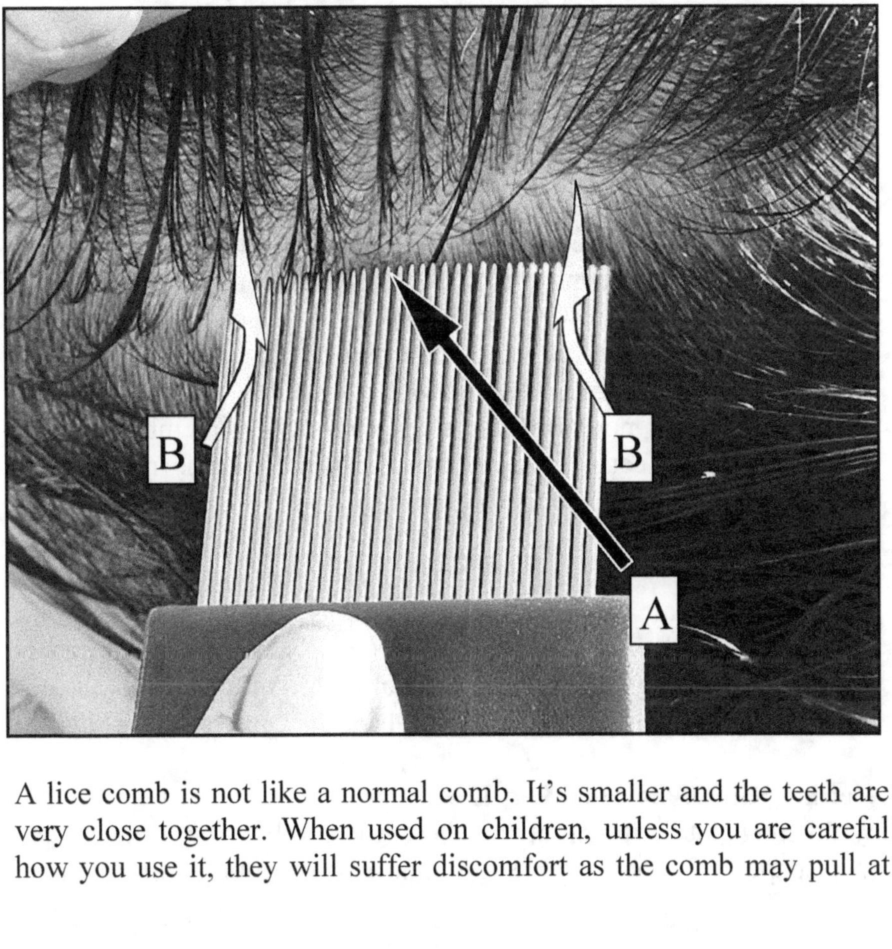

B   B   A

A lice comb is not like a normal comb. It's smaller and the teeth are very close together. When used on children, unless you are careful how you use it, they will suffer discomfort as the comb may pull at their hair if used incorrectly.

The right way is to divide their hair up into manageable tufts. A good system is to start from the back and then move forwards up and over the top and sides, separating the hair into portions as you go. You comb from the root to the tip. Its good to have a saucer or small bowl of water close by to dip the comb into and some tissues to keep wiping the comb into the water after each comb stroke.

You can lightly wash the hair in a mild shampoo and comb it whilst wet so the comb slips more readily through the hair.
[A]: Position the comb carefully at the root of the hair tuft.
[B]: Insert the comb and sweep it upwards until it leaves the tufts of hair at their tips.

Looking After Your Comb

You are going to be using the comb over a period of 21 days, maybe on more than one person, like the whole family. It is going to encounter the odd hair knot. The gaps between the teeth are likely to change if the individual teeth distort or bend sideways. You can use a small screw driver or the tip of a nail file to gently ease them all straight again. Always check the comb. *Gaps mean escaping lice!*

Disinfection?

There is actually no need to disinfect to comb in relation to the lice. But, you might accidently ping the scalp of someone being lice-combed and this can in very rare instances introduce bacteria into the scalp. So, you can soak the comb in a diluted disinfecting agent over night and wash it before combing. We use Dettol, a brand name, in the UK. There is no desire to have your family members' heads smelling of disinfectant, so put the comb under some running tap water before starting to comb.

Hair Washing

Washing your hair too often can lead to washing out important oils, vital for the health and balance of your hair's condition. Instead of combing wet hair, you can use a little atomiser spray, and spray each tuft of hair lightly as you go. This will help the comb slide through.

Getting Rid Of Combed Out Lice

With long hair, it might be best to comb over some paper (newspaper?) laid on a table top. You can sit your family member down and let them bend their head over the table and paper. This way, any lice not staying on the comb fall onto the paper. When you are finished, simple gather the paper up into a scrunched ball and put it into the trash.

Misconceptions

People say they have combed lice eggs out. They haven't. You can't. What they are seeing are the dried out skins moulted by younger lice as they grew bigger. They leave the skins behind. This happens several times.

Vital

All members of a household or family must be combed on the same day, preferably during a similar period of time. This is to ensure cross-infestation is minimised.

Chapter 4: The Program

This is the main thing you have to do. Many knowledgeable people will offer advice about how to get rid of head lice. Some of that advice will involve the combing 'idea'. And this is the problem. An idea! So it snows, and two people, your friends, mention how to clear the snow from the path. One idea is use salt. The other suggestion is to shovel it away. Salt seems easier. No hard work. We do that. It doesn't work. We needed a lot more salt than we thought. We try the shovel. We buy a cheap shovel and we get to work. But as we get half way through, it snows again. God! We look back... covered again.

Combing without a routine and a worked out method is just like that. You can use the chemicals. They don't work. You can just comb away, without any system. That won't work either.

The problem is the new lice are very tiny indeed. You will not even be able to see them in the hair with the naked eye. Combing will certainly get out the larger more mature lice, and it may seem for a week or two, you have cleared them. But those tiny, wee lice which slipped easily through spaced between the comb teeth will be growing and soon, they will be mature enough to mate and lay more impossible-to-remove eggs. And there will be eggs reaching hatching stage left behind from the lice you combed out.

What the Lice Program does is apply a knowledge of when the

eggs will hatch, and when baby lice left behind will reach maturity and can mate and lay eggs. Fortunately, there are critical days when all the eggs have hatched and critical days where newly mature lice are around but can't mate yet. So, if we remove all the active mature lice first, and then remove the smaller ones when they get a bit bigger and before they can mate, and then wait for any and all remaining eggs to hatch, and the new young to grow big enough, we can get all the lice out with none left to start another generation. And this... if I may repeat myself because it is an absolute truth... This is the only way to get rid of lice effectively, side-effect free, and with no risks to people or children that might be caused through the use of unknown chemical treatments.

This works!

The 21 days of your program on the opposite page enable you to see and check each day and what you need to do for a short time that day. Any marked in GREY mean you don't need to take any action at all that day, so you and your family can have a normal evening. **Be careful though that your** GREY **days of rest do not cause laziness or complacency: the battle will not be won unless you follow the Program Exactly!**

There are 13 days in the whole 21 days when you actually have to do something. These are marked with asterisks (little stars) to the right of each day. Four stars means critical. Two stars mean Very Important. All the days filled in with light grey are lazy days: nothing to do lice-wise!

The VIP days are days number: 0 (the day you start, day 5, day 12, day 16, and day 21.

The other lice combing days are: day 1(the day after the day you start), day 2, day 7, day 9, day 14, day 15, day 19, and day 20.

You won't have to remember these because I have put 21 pages into this book which you can use to keep a record of what days you comb and any issues you need to remember.

Identify your stage
in the 21 day program

Not started yet ->   **Start Here**

Entering the war->	**Day 0 VIP**	****
Removing the Layers->	Day 1	**
Getting the evaders->	Day 2	**
Re-arming (Rest)->	Day 3	
Re-arming (Rest)->	Day 4	
Final Sweep 1->	**Day 5 VIP**	****
Re-arming (Rest)->	Day 6	
Facing their 2nd attack->	Day 7	**
Re-arming (Rest)->	Day 8	
Getting the 2nd Wave->	Day 9	**
Re-arming (Rest)->	Day 10	
Re-arming (Rest)->	Day 11	
Final Sweep 2->	**Day 12 VIP**	****
Re-arming (Rest)->	Day 13	
Critical Action a->	Day 14	**
Critical Action b->	Day 15	**
Super-Critical Day->	**Day 16 VIP**	****
Re-arming (Rest)->	Day 17	
Re-arming (Rest)->	Day 18	
Belt & Braces day 1->	Day 19	**
Belt & Braces day 2->	Day 20	**
Last Chance Day->	**Day 21 VIP**	****

Program Over

This is the program for ...

_____

_____

_____

_____

_____

_____

Started: _____

Planned end date: _____
(21 days later).

DAY 0 - Date : _____

What day of the week is it? Mark it below by ringing the day with a pen.

Sun   **Mon**   **Tue**   **Wed**

Thur   **Fri**   **Sat**

VIP DAY. MUST COMB TODAY!

Names of everyone to be combed. And the time of day they are going to be combed. Tick when they are!

Name	Time	Done
_____	_____	☐
_____	_____	☐
_____	_____	☐
_____	_____	☐
_____	_____	☐
_____	_____	☐
_____	_____	☐
_____	_____	☐
_____	_____	☐

Notes:

DAY 1 - Date : _____

What day of the week is it? Mark it below by ringing the day with a pen.

Sun	Mon	Tue	Wed
Thur		Fri	Sat

MUST COMB TODAY!

Names of everyone to be combed. And the time of day they are going to be combed. Tick when they are!

Name	Time	Done
_____	_____	☐
_____	_____	☐
_____	_____	☐
_____	_____	☐
_____	_____	☐
_____	_____	☐
_____	_____	☐
_____	_____	☐
_____	_____	☐

Notes:

DAY 2 - Date :

What day of the week is it? Mark it below by ringing the day with a pen.

Sun   Mon   Tue   Wed

Thur   Fri   Sat

MUST COMB TODAY!

Names of everyone to be combed. And the time of day they are going to be combed. Tick when they are!

Name	Time	Done
_____	_____	☐
_____	_____	☐
_____	_____	☐
_____	_____	☐
_____	_____	☐
_____	_____	☐
_____	_____	☐
_____	_____	☐
_____	_____	☐

Notes:

DAY 3 - Date :

What day of the week is it? Mark it below by ringing the day with a pen.

Sun	**Mon**	**Tue**	**Wed**
Thur	**Fri**	**Sat**	

Names of everyone to be ~~combed. And the time of day they are going to~~ **NO COMBING DAY!** ~~when they are!~~

Name	Time	Done
_____	_____	☐
_____	_____	☐
_____	_____	☐
_____	_____	☐
_____	_____	☐
_____	_____	☐
_____	_____	☐
_____	_____	☐
_____	_____	☐

Notes:

DAY 4 - Date :

What day of the week is it? Mark it below by ringing the day with a pen.

Sun	Mon	Tue	Wed
Thur		Fri	Sat

NO COMBING DAY!

Names of everyone to be combed and the time of day they are going to be combed and when they are!

Name	Time	Done
_____	_____	☐
_____	_____	☐
_____	_____	☐
_____	_____	☐
_____	_____	☐
_____	_____	☐
_____	_____	☐
_____	_____	☐
_____	_____	☐

Notes:

DAY 5 - Date : _____

What day of the week is it? Mark it below by ringing the day with a pen.

Sun	Mon	Tue	Wed

Thur　　　**Fri**　　　**Sat**

VIP DAY. MUST COMB TODAY!

Names of everyone to be combed. And the time of day they are going to be combed. Tick when they are!

Name	Time	Done
_____	_____	☐
_____	_____	☐
_____	_____	☐
_____	_____	☐
_____	_____	☐
_____	_____	☐
_____	_____	☐
_____	_____	☐
_____	_____	☐

Notes:

DAY 6 - Date :

What day of the week is it? Mark it below by ringing the day with a pen.

Sun	Mon	Tue	Wed
Thur		Fri	Sat

Names of everyone to be combing the time of day they are going to be combed and when they are!

NO COMBING DAY!

Name	Time	Done
_____	_____	☐
_____	_____	☐
_____	_____	☐
_____	_____	☐
_____	_____	☐
_____	_____	☐
_____	_____	☐
_____	_____	☐
_____	_____	☐

Notes:

DAY 7 - Date :

What day of the week is it? Mark it below by ringing the day with a pen.

Sun   Mon   Tue   Wed

Thur   Fri   Sat

MUST COMB TODAY!

Names of everyone to be combed. And the time of day they are going to be combed. Tick when they are!

Name	Time	Done
_____	_____	☐
_____	_____	☐
_____	_____	☐
_____	_____	☐
_____	_____	☐
_____	_____	☐
_____	_____	☐
_____	_____	☐
_____	_____	☐

Notes:

DAY 8 - Date :

What day of the week is it? Mark it below by ringing the day with a pen.

Sun	Mon	Tue	Wed

Thur	Fri	Sat

Names of everyone to ~~be~~ ~~combing~~ ~~the~~ time of day they are goi~~ng~~ ~~to~~ ~~be~~ ~~combed~~ ~~tick~~ when they are!

NO COMBING DAY!

Name	Time	Done
_____	_____	☐
_____	_____	☐
_____	_____	☐
_____	_____	☐
_____	_____	☐
_____	_____	☐
_____	_____	☐
_____	_____	☐
_____	_____	☐

Notes:

DAY 9 - Date : _____

What day of the week is it? Mark it below by ringing the day with a pen.

Sun	Mon	Tue	Wed

Thur	Fri	Sat

MUST COMB TODAY!

Names of everyone to be combed. And the time of day they are going to be combed. Tick when they are!

Name	Time	Done
_____	_____	☐
_____	_____	☐
_____	_____	☐
_____	_____	☐
_____	_____	☐
_____	_____	☐
_____	_____	☐
_____	_____	☐
_____	_____	☐

Notes:

DAY 10 - Date :

What day of the week is it? Mark it below by ringing the day with a pen.

Sun	Mon	Tue	Wed

Thur   **Fri**   **Sat**

NO COMBING DAY!

Names of everyone to ~~be~~ ~~~~ the time of day they are goi~~ng to~~ be co~~mbed a~~nd when they are!

Name	Time	Done
_____	_____	☐
_____	_____	☐
_____	_____	☐
_____	_____	☐
_____	_____	☐
_____	_____	☐
_____	_____	☐
_____	_____	☐
_____	_____	☐

Notes:

DAY 11 - Date :

What day of the week is it? Mark it below by ringing the day with a pen.

Sun	Mon	Tue	Wed

Thur	Fri	Sat

NO COMBING DAY!

Names of everyone to be combed and the time of day they are going to be combed. Tick when they are!

Name	Time	Done
_____	_____	☐
_____	_____	☐
_____	_____	☐
_____	_____	☐
_____	_____	☐
_____	_____	☐
_____	_____	☐
_____	_____	☐
_____	_____	☐

Notes:

DAY 12 -   Date :

What day of the week is it? Mark it below by ringing the day with a pen.

Sun	**Mon**	**Tue**	**Wed**
Thur	**Fri**	**Sat**	

VIP DAY. MUST COMB TODAY!

Names of everyone to be combed. And the time of day they are going to be combed. Tick when they are!

Name	Time	Done
_____	_____	☐
_____	_____	☐
_____	_____	☐
_____	_____	☐
_____	_____	☐
_____	_____	☐
_____	_____	☐
_____	_____	☐
_____	_____	☐

Notes:

DAY 13 - Date :

What day of the week is it? Mark it below by ringing the day with a pen.

Sun   **Mon**   **Tue**   **Wed**

Thur   **Fri**   **Sat**

NO COMBING DAY!

Names of everyone to ~~be combed~~ **and the time of day they are g**~~oing to be combed.~~ **Tick when they are!**

Name	Time	Done
_____	_____	☐
_____	_____	☐
_____	_____	☐
_____	_____	☐
_____	_____	☐
_____	_____	☐
_____	_____	☐
_____	_____	☐
_____	_____	☐

Notes:

DAY 14 -   Date :

What day of the week is it? Mark it below by ringing the day with a pen.

Sun   Mon   Tue   Wed

Thur   Fri   Sat

MUST COMB TODAY!

Names of everyone to be combed. And the time of day they are going to be combed. Tick when they are!

Name	Time	Done
_____	_____	☐
_____	_____	☐
_____	_____	☐
_____	_____	☐
_____	_____	☐
_____	_____	☐
_____	_____	☐
_____	_____	☐
_____	_____	☐

Notes:

DAY 15 - Date : _____

What day of the week is it? Mark it below by ringing the day with a pen.

Sun	Mon	Tue	Wed

Thur	Fri	Sat

MUST COMB TODAY!

Names of everyone to be combed. And the time of day they are going to be combed. Tick when they are!

Name	Time	Done
_____	_____	☐
_____	_____	☐
_____	_____	☐
_____	_____	☐
_____	_____	☐
_____	_____	☐
_____	_____	☐
_____	_____	☐
_____	_____	☐

Notes:

DAY 16 -Date :

What day of the week is it? Mark it below by ringing the day with a pen.

Sun	Mon	Tue	Wed

Thur   **Fri**   **Sat**

VIP DAY. MUST COMB TODAY!

Names of everyone to be combed. And the time of day they are going to be combed. Tick when they are!

Name	Time	Done
_____	_____	☐
_____	_____	☐
_____	_____	☐
_____	_____	☐
_____	_____	☐
_____	_____	☐
_____	_____	☐
_____	_____	☐
_____	_____	☐

Notes:

DAY 17 -   Date :

What day of the week is it? Mark it below by ringing the day with a pen.

Sun	**Mon**	**Tue**	**Wed**
Thur	**Fri**	**Sat**	

NO COMBING DAY!

Names of everyone to be combing the name of **day they are going** be combing **when they are!**

Name	Time	Done
_____	_____	☐
_____	_____	☐
_____	_____	☐
_____	_____	☐
_____	_____	☐
_____	_____	☐
_____	_____	☐
_____	_____	☐
_____	_____	☐

Notes:

DAY 18 -   Date :

What day of the week is it? Mark it below by ringing the day with a pen.

Sun   **Mon**   **Tue**   **Wed**

Thur   **Fri**   **Sat**

NO COMBING DAY!

Names of everyone to be combed and the time of day they are going to be combed. Tick when they are!

Name	Time	Done
_____	_____	☐
_____	_____	☐
_____	_____	☐
_____	_____	☐
_____	_____	☐
_____	_____	☐
_____	_____	☐
_____	_____	☐
_____	_____	☐

Notes:

DAY 19 -   Date :

What day of the week is it? Mark it below by ringing the day with a pen.

Sun	Mon	Tue	Wed

Thur	Fri	Sat

MUST COMB TODAY!

Names of everyone to be combed. And the time of day they are going to be combed. Tick when they are!

Name	Time	Done
_____	_____	☐
_____	_____	☐
_____	_____	☐
_____	_____	☐
_____	_____	☐
_____	_____	☐
_____	_____	☐
_____	_____	☐
_____	_____	☐

Notes:

DAY 20 -   Date :

What day of the week is it? Mark it below by ringing the day with a pen.

Sun   Mon   Tue   Wed

Thur   Fri   Sat

MUST COMB TODAY!

Names of everyone to be combed. And the time of day they are going to be combed. Tick when they are!

Name	Time	Done
_____	_____	☐
_____	_____	☐
_____	_____	☐
_____	_____	☐
_____	_____	☐
_____	_____	☐
_____	_____	☐
_____	_____	☐
_____	_____	☐

Notes:

DAY 21 -   Date :   _____

What day of the week is it? Mark it below by ringing the day with a pen.

Sun   Mon   Tue   Wed

Thur   Fri   Sat

VIP DAY. MUST COMB TODAY!

Names of everyone to be combed. And the time of day they are going to be combed. Tick when they are!

Name	Time	Done
_____	_____	☐
_____	_____	☐
_____	_____	☐
_____	_____	☐
_____	_____	☐
_____	_____	☐
_____	_____	☐
_____	_____	☐
_____	_____	☐

Notes:

FINISHED!
LICE
GONE!

Chapter 4: Staying Lice-free

Finally, the lice are gone! The hard work is over. You can relax. Except, well... you have to make sure your family, especially young children, remain free of lice. This, unfortunately, does take a little bit more of extra work. It is only when you have young children. Lice seem to love children who have not yet reached their teenage years. No one is certain why.

Young children have habits of hugging or behaviour which might bring their heads in slight contact when at play, in school. It's highly likely that one or more of the other children in the class your child goes to is also infested. And this is how the lice continue to flourish. Mums and dads clear the infestation in their own children, often discreetly, but because some other child's mum or dad hasn't noticed the lice problem with their child yet, the de-loused child is likely to pick up lice again from the infested one.

There are two things you can do. You need to be brave and forthright to do it, and not appear accusational at all. The first is you could contact the teacher in your child's class and suggest they prepare a small friendly note for kids to give their parents. I have put an example on the opposite page.

The second is to tell your child not to put their head near another kid's head. I wouldn't do that with very young children. It sends out the wrong message to them about mixing and being at one with others. Maybe with older children, you can do this?

If you are close to any of the other parents of children in the same class as your one, you could have a friendly chat and ask them to spread the information, such that other parents check their kids for lice. The choice is up to you, but if you do nothing, and you have young children, it is likely they will get lice all over again.

And just to help myself, as well as all those other families, you could mention this book to other parents, or get the school to buy one so that the information can be understood easily by others in the future. If they wish to check out the web site, it's:

www.microscopy-uk.org.uk/heliceprogram/

It is now a recommended method of clearing lice by Berkerely Education.

See here:

http://parents.berkeley.edu/advice/health/lice.html

Example letter for teachers to give parents.

Teachers Name
Class Name / number
School Name
Date: School Address

Dear Parent,

A few cases or hair lice infestation have been noted in the class. Fortunately, the parents were on the case and have taken steps to clear this up. But, it may be best for each parent to do a check on their children so we can all be assured we are not bothered with this for long.

Just to say, hair lice do **not** cause any health problems for children or adults, but are just not very nice to have. Lice love clean hair and young children's heads. And every now and then, most schools, seem to have a lot of cases of them, before it settles down again for a few years.

Various treatments can be purchased inexpensively to eradicate hair lice, but we are not positioned to suggest one method over another. A quick look-up on-line (the internet) can provide additional information.

Many thanks for your help and support with this minor nuisance.

Sincerely,

Teacher's name.

And that is about it. I know if you use the program as recommended here, you will get rid of the lice. But you might not be able to get to comb everyone on the same day, which tends to weaken the effectiveness of the program. But, you might, just might get away with it. Everyone in the household (family) should be combed, not just the kids, and not just anyone found with hair lice in the family. All of the family must be combed. Ideally, on the same day, and although never normally possible, at the same time of day.

I hope I have helped you. I know the nuisance lice cause and the way it starts to take over your life. No-one wants that. Life is for living and aiming to have a full and pleasant experience. And with that, and my genuine warmth, I sign off for now.

Mol Smith
Author of The Lice Program.